AF270691

MY FRIEND WITH ASTHMA

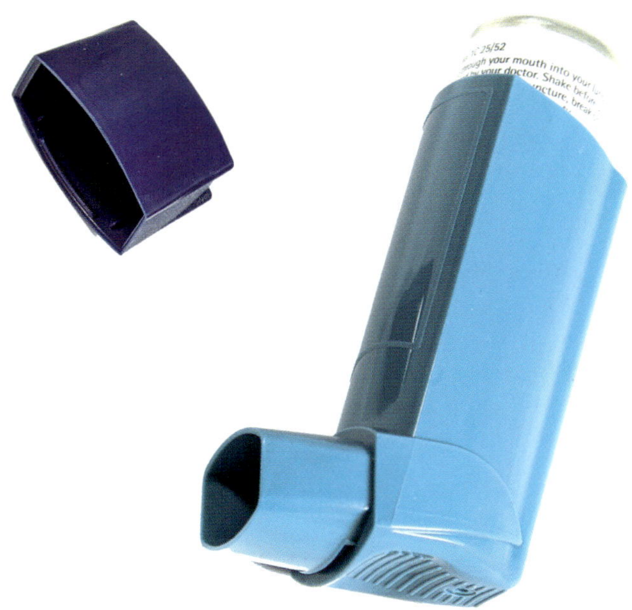

by Elizabeth Andrews

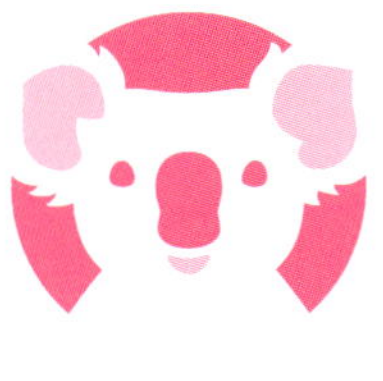

Cody Koala
An Imprint of Pop!
popbooksonline.com

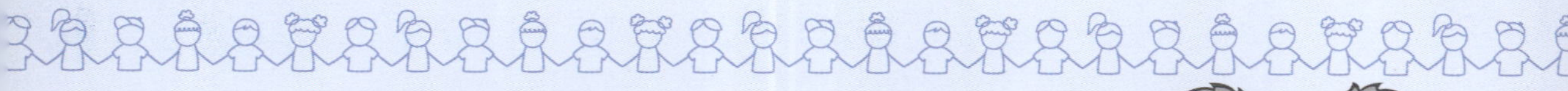

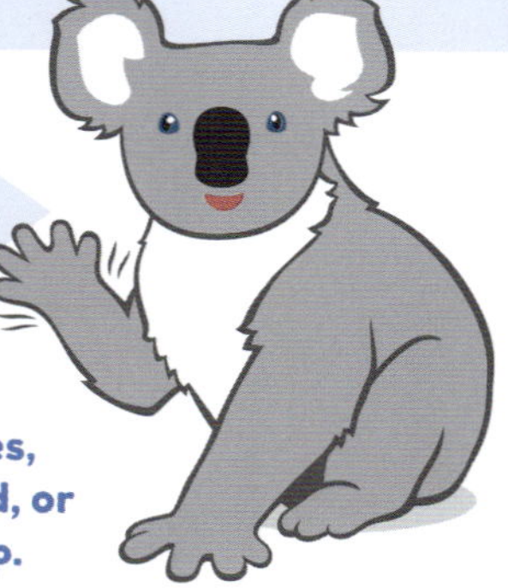

This book is filled with videos, puzzles, games, and more! Scan the QR codes* while you read, or visit the website below to make this book pop.

popbooksonline.com/asthma

*Scanning QR codes requires a web-enabled smart device with a QR code reader app and a camera.

abdobooks.com

Published by Pop!, a division of ABDO, PO Box 398166, Minneapolis, Minnesota 55439. Copyright ©2024 by Abdo Consulting Group, Inc. International copyrights reserved in all countries. No part of this book may be reproduced in any form without written permission from the publisher. Cody Koala™ is a trademark and logo of Pop!.

Printed in the United States of America, North Mankato, Minnesota.

102023
012024

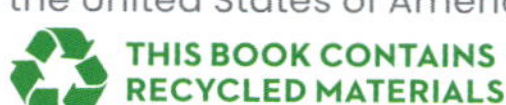
THIS BOOK CONTAINS
RECYCLED MATERIALS

Cover Photo: Shutterstock Images
Interior Photos: Shutterstock Images; Getty Images
Editor: Grace Hansen
Series Designer: Victoria Bates

Library of Congress Control Number: 2023938795

Publisher's Cataloging-in-Publication Data
Names: Andrews, Elizabeth, author.
Title: My friend with asthma / by Elizabeth Andrews
Description: Minneapolis, Minnesota : Pop!, 2024 | Series: My friend with health needs | Includes online resources and index
Identifiers: ISBN 9781098245290 (lib. bdg.) | ISBN 9781098245856 (ebook)
Subjects: LCSH: Friendship--Juvenile literature. | Asthma--Juvenile literature. | Asthmatics--Juvenile literature. | Social acceptance--Juvenile literature.
Classification: DDC 616.24--dc23

Table of Contents

Chapter 1

Breathing Safely

Peter is running the mile in PE class today. Before class, he stops by the nurse's office to use his **inhaler**. Peter has asthma. Using his inhaler means he can run the mile safely.

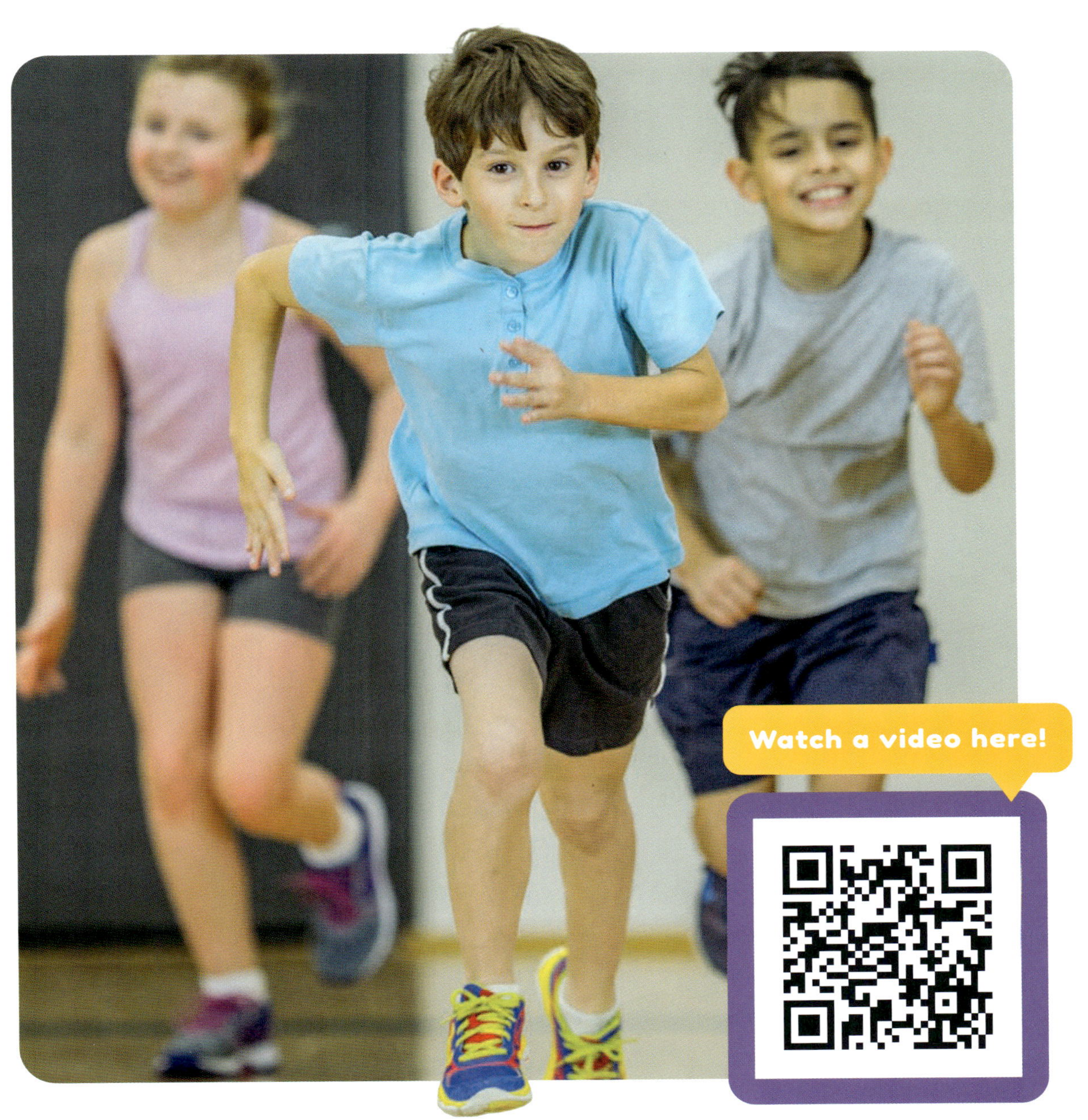
Watch a video here!

Chapter 2

What Is Asthma?

Asthma makes breathing difficult. People breathe air into their **lungs** through their nose and mouth. The air travels through pipes called airways.

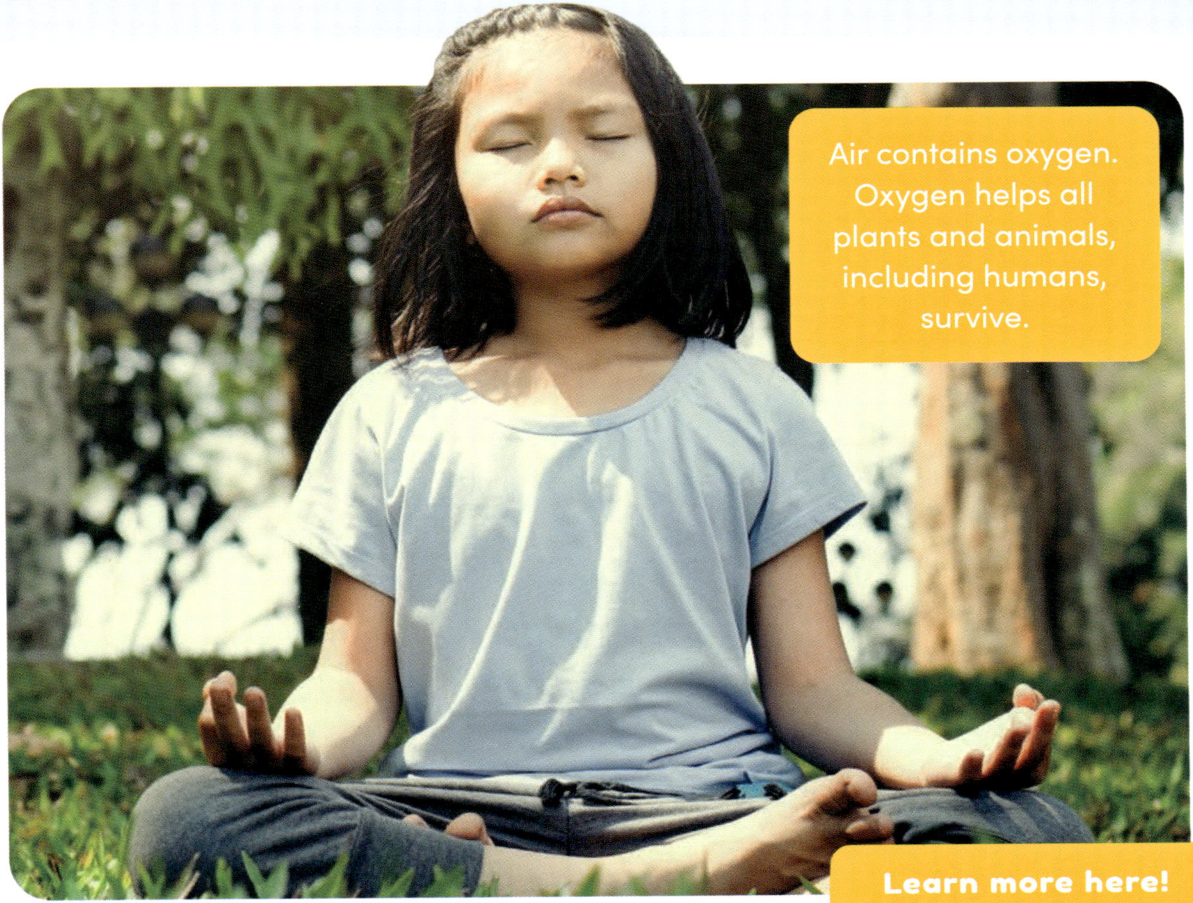

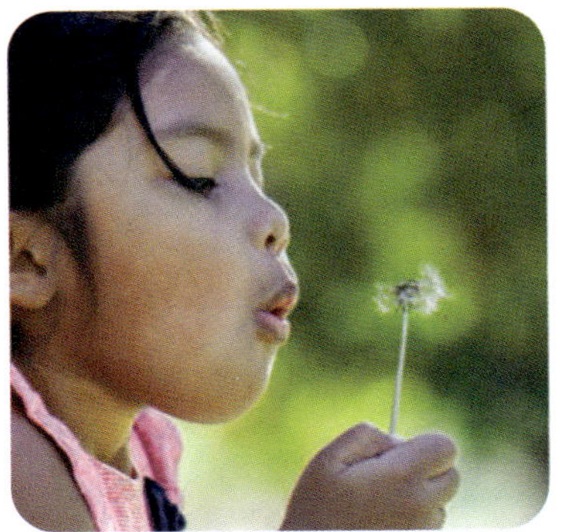
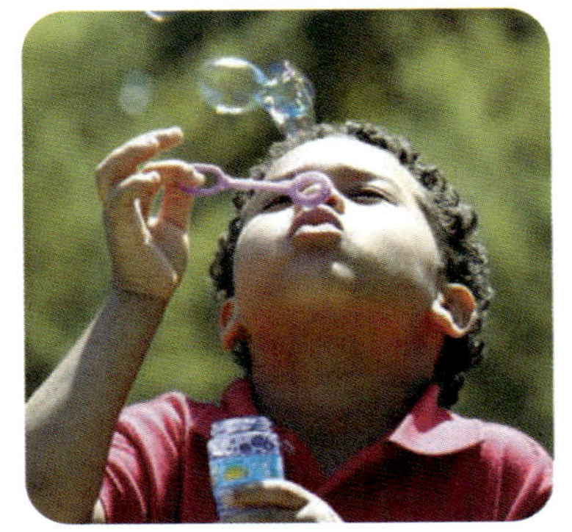

Air contains oxygen. Oxygen helps all plants and animals, including humans, survive.
Learn more here!

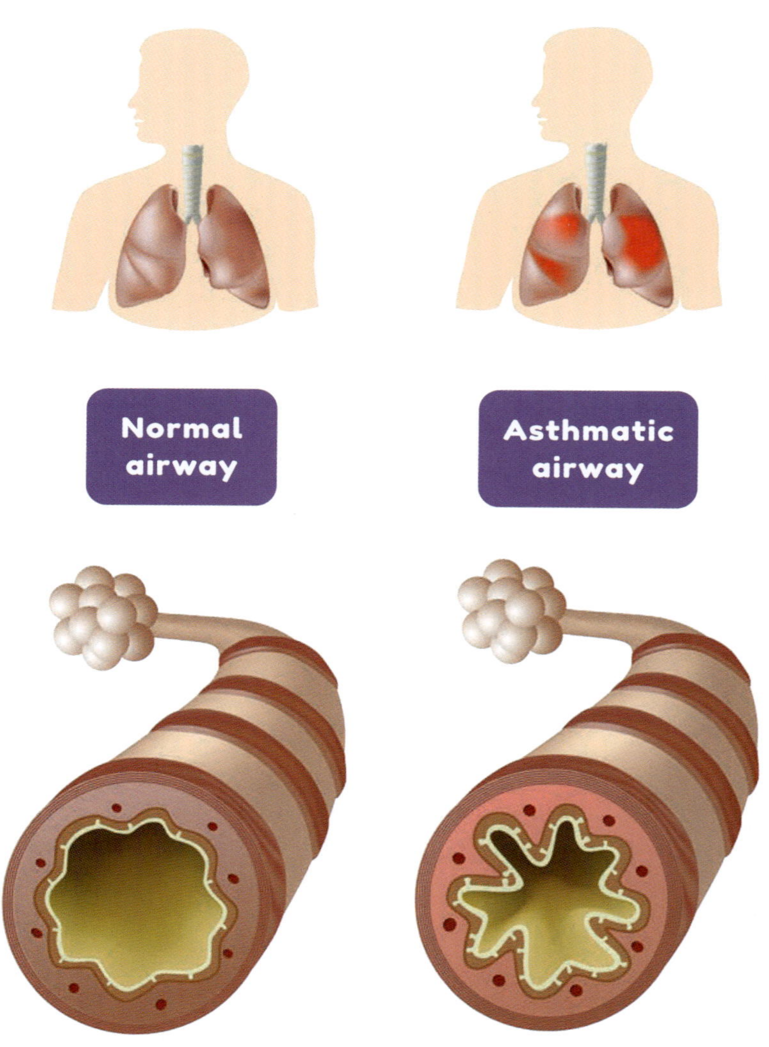

Normal
airway
Asthmatic
airway

People with asthma have airways that are **swollen** and tighter than they should be. With smaller airways, it is harder for air to flow through. This can make the chest feel tight and cause **wheezing**.

Airways swell for different reasons. Breathing in smoke, chemicals, or **allergens** can cause swelling. Exercise and cold air may cause it too. People with asthma try to **avoid** these things.

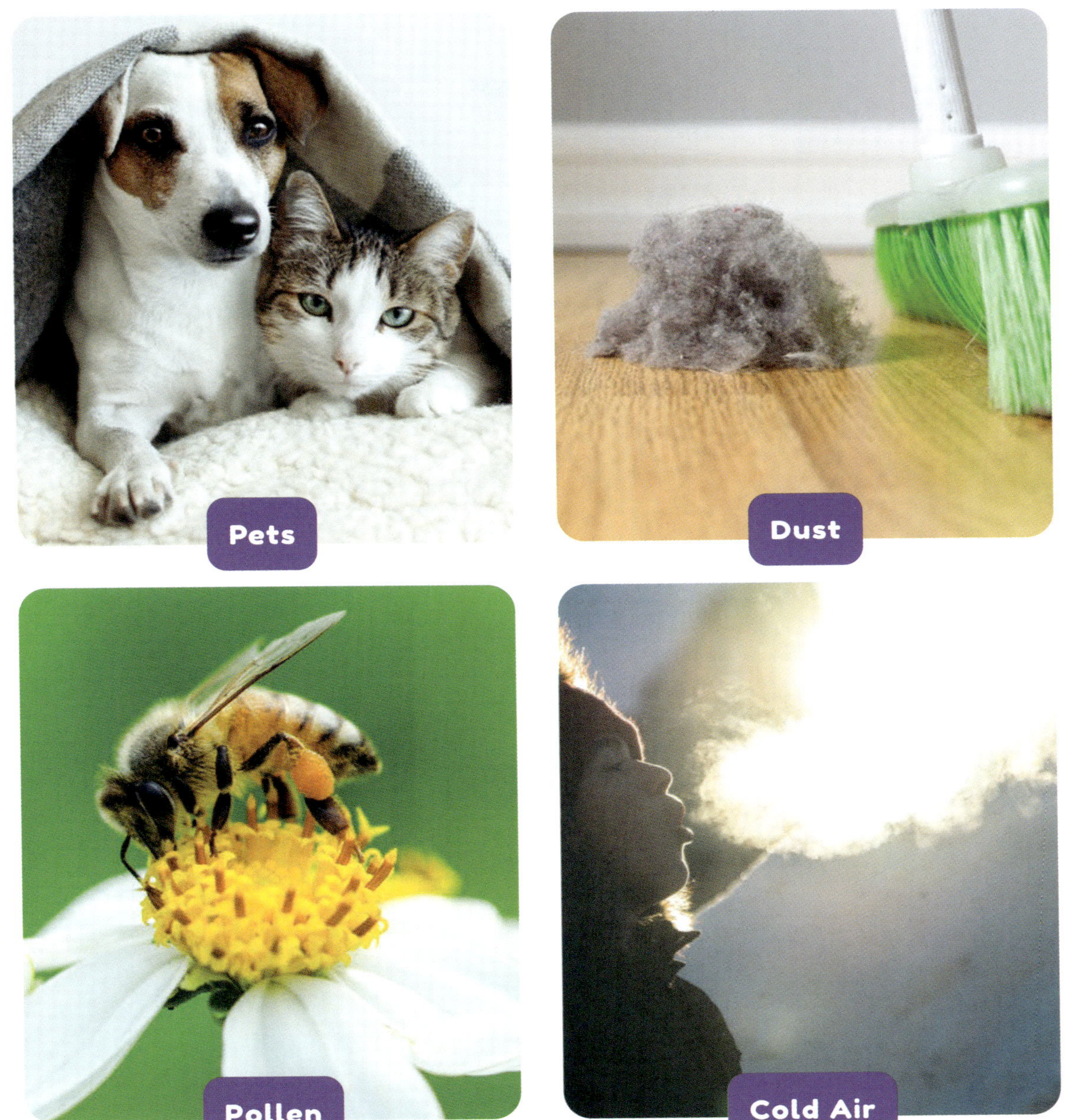

Pets
Dust
Pollen
Cold Air

Chapter 3

Taking Care of Asthma

An asthma attack happens when a person's airway gets too tight to allow air through. They will cough and **wheeze**. Their heart beats fast.

Some people use inhalers every day. Inhalers contain medicine that helps open the airway.

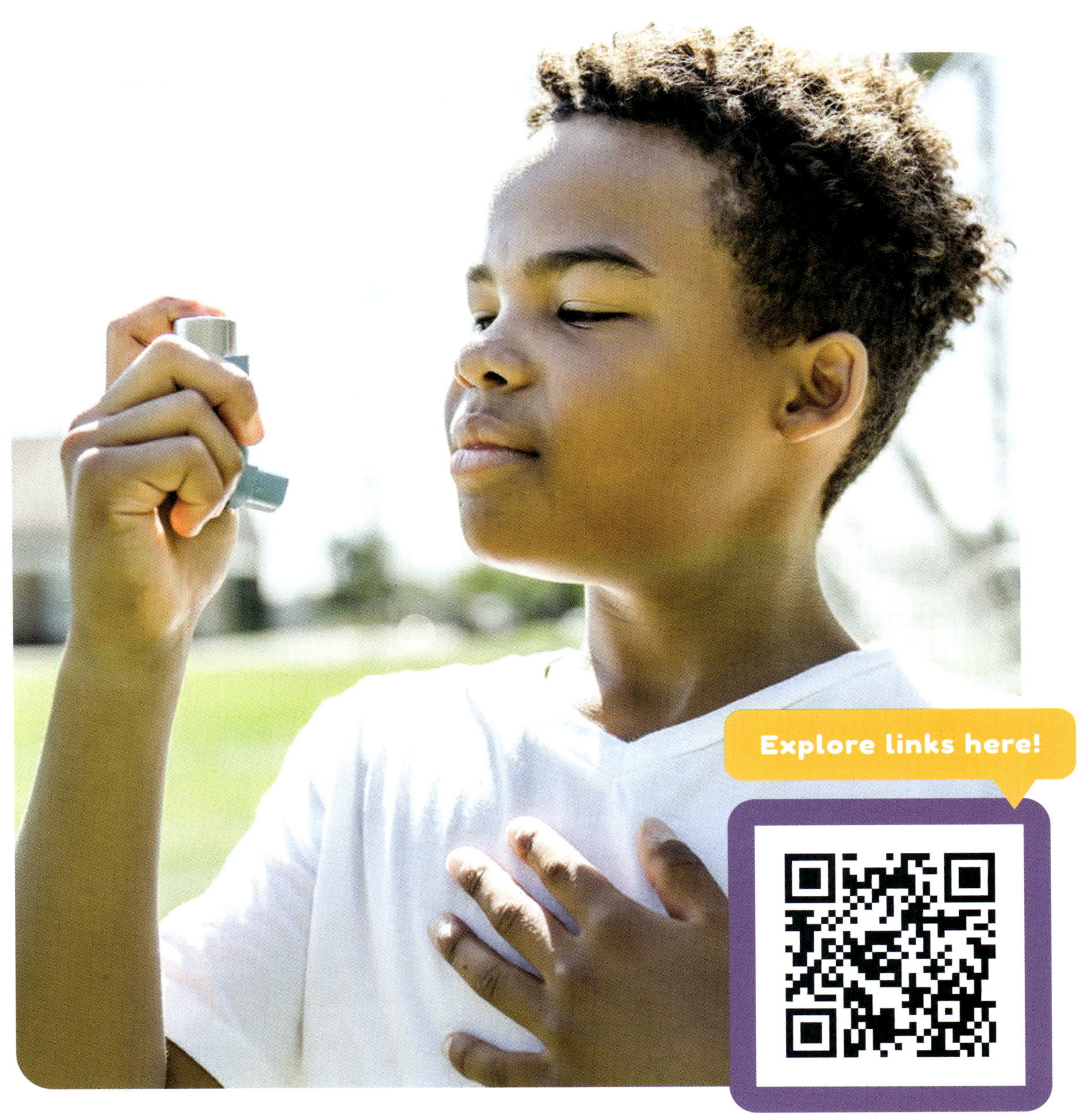
Explore links here!

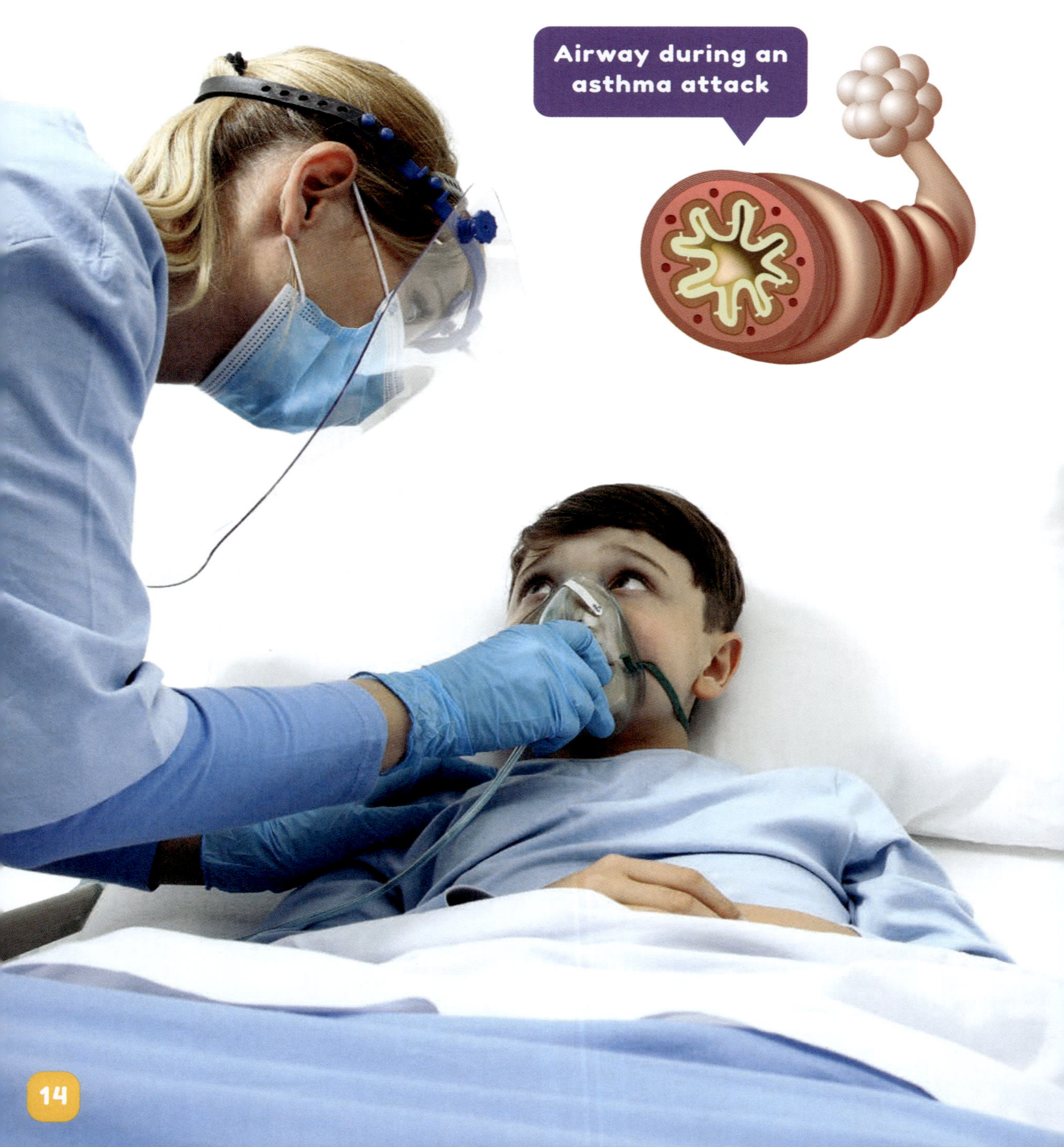
Airway during an
asthma attack

An asthma attack can last from a few minutes to several hours. People use **inhalers** to stop an attack. However, if an asthma attack is bad enough, a person needs to go to the hospital.

Children with asthma create a plan with their doctor and **guardian** to help care for their asthma. A plan explains which medicines to take and **triggers** to **avoid**. It also explains when it's time to go to the hospital.

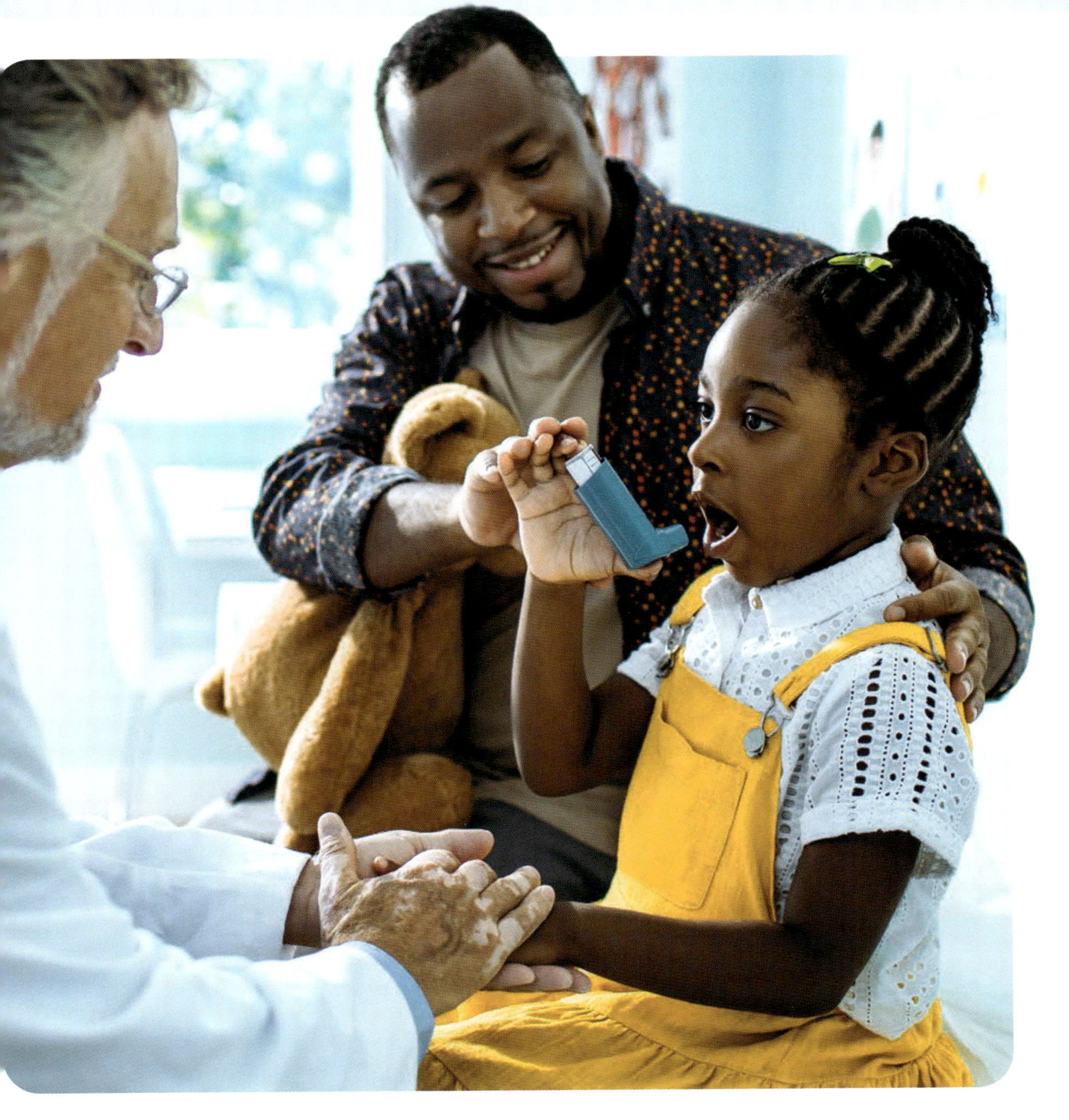

Chapter 4

Growing with Asthma

People can get asthma at any age. It is most common in children because their airways are smaller. It may get better as a child grows because their airways grow larger too.

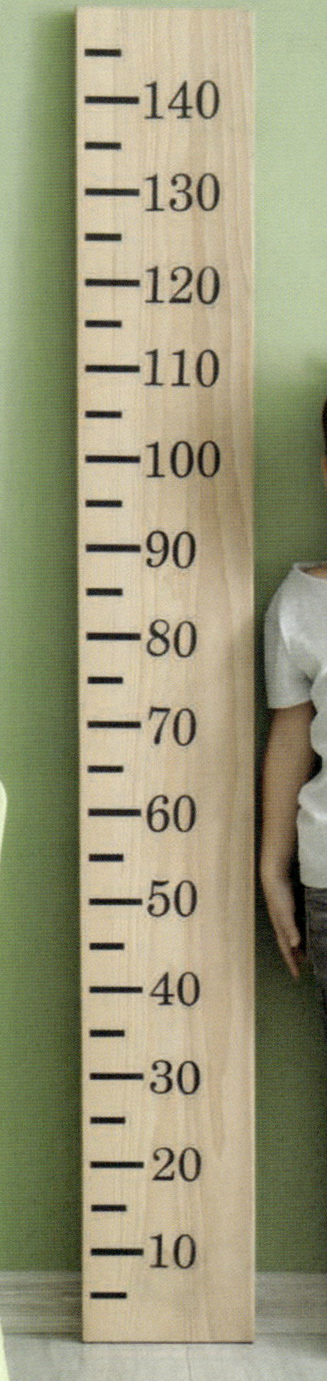

140
130
120
110
100
90
80
70
60
50
40
30
20
10

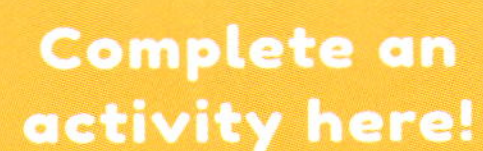

Complete an
activity here!

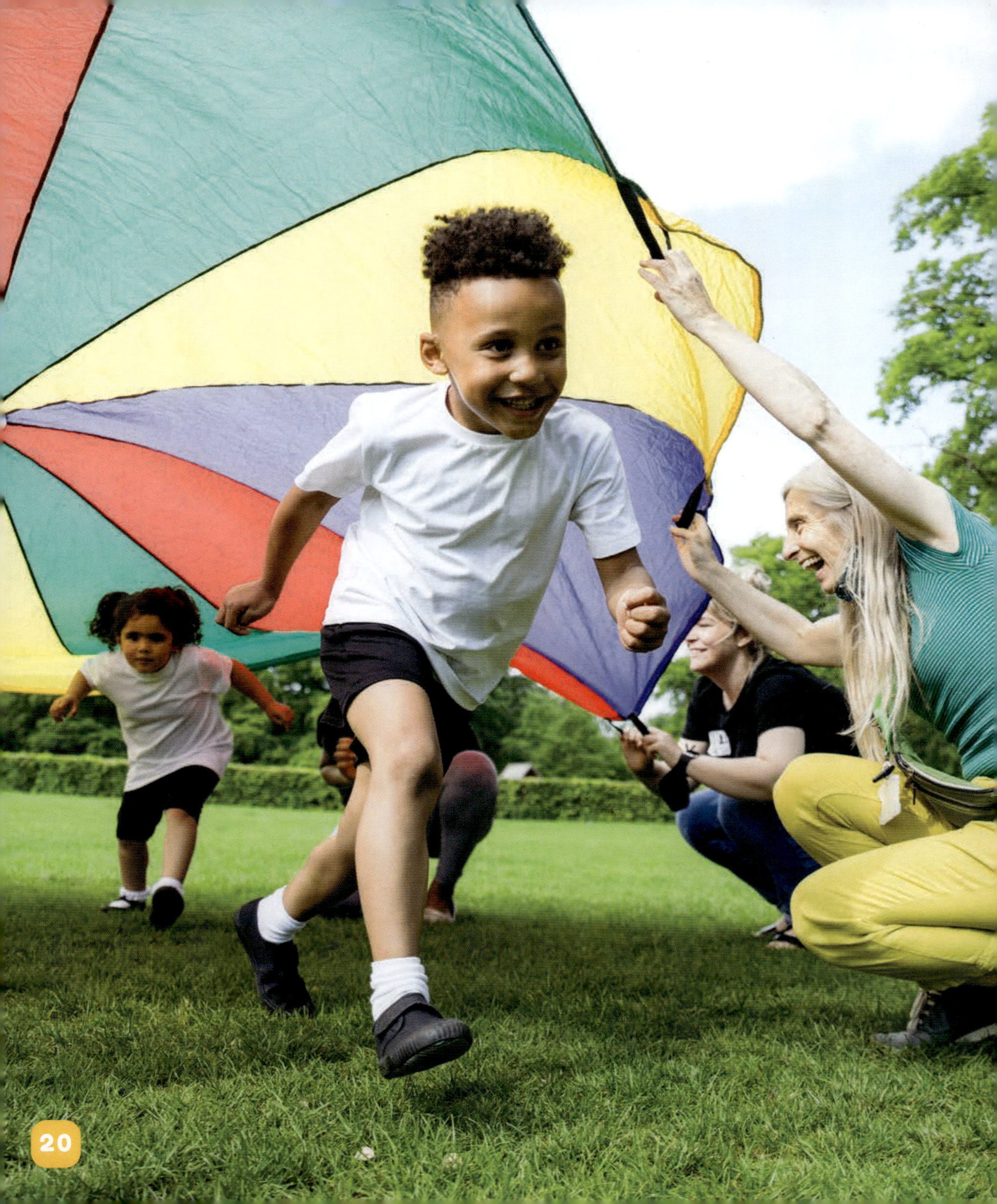

Millions of children have asthma. Everyone's asthma is different. As long as a person is taking care of their asthma, they can usually do anything they dream of.

Making Connections

Text-to-Self

Do you or any of your friends have asthma? What is having asthma like for you or them?

Text-to-Text

Have you read any other books about people with health needs? How were those needs similar to or different from asthma?

Text-to-World

Do you think going outside helps or hurts people with asthma? How do you think people with asthma prepare for outdoor activities?

Glossary

allergen – something breathed in that can cause asthma symptoms.

avoid – to keep away from.

guardian – an adult chosen by law to be responsible for the care and protection of a child.

inhaler – a device that releases medicine as a mist meant to be breathed in.

lungs – a pair of body parts in the chest that fill with air and pass on oxygen to the blood.

swell – (*verb*) to grow beyond normal size. (*noun*) the act or process of swelling.

trigger – to cause or set off.

wheeze – to breathe with difficulty usually with a whistling sound.

Index

Online Resources

popbooksonline.com

Thanks for reading this Cody Koala book!

This book is filled with videos, puzzles, games, and more! Scan the QR codes* while you read, or visit the website below to make this book pop.

popbooksonline.com/asthma

*Scanning QR codes requires a web-enabled smart device with a QR code reader app and a camera.